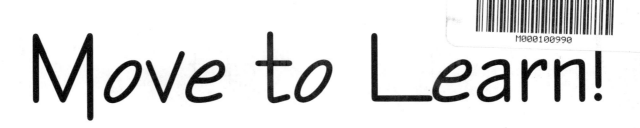

Move to Learn!

Games and Incentives to Reinforce Content Learning

Written by Nadine Rogers and Tina West

Illustrated by Vanessa Countryman

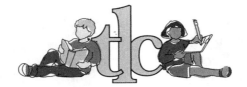

Teaching & Learning Company

1204 Buchanan St., P.O. Box 10
Carthage, IL 62321-0010

This book belongs to

_____

Cover art by Vanessa Countryman

Cover design by Jenny Morgan

Copyright © 2008, Teaching & Learning Company

ISBN No. 10: 1-57310-560-0

ISBN No. 13: 978-1-57310-560-6

Printing No. 987654321

Teaching & Learning Company
1204 Buchanan St., P.O. Box 10
Carthage, IL 62321-0010

The purchase of this book entitles teachers to make copies for use in their individual classrooms only. This book, or any part of it, may not be reproduced in any form for any other purposes without prior written permission from the Teaching & Learning Company. It is strictly prohibited to reproduce any part of this book for an entire school or school district, or for commercial resale. The above permission is exclusive of the cover art, which may not be reproduced.

All rights reserved. Printed in the United States of America.

TLC10560 Copyright © Teaching & Learning Company, Carthage, IL 62321-0010

Table of Contents

The Importance of Movement in Learning

Today's brain, mind and body research establishes links between movement and learning. Neurologists think people are born with the number of brain cells they will have. A person doesn't produce new brain cells, therefore you must increase the number of the connections between neurons to become capable of complex ways of thinking.

Scientists have found that moving the body maximizes brain power and increases the connections between neurons. Even a simple movement can bring about improvement in a child's memory and concentration levels. This is why activity in the classroom is so important in teaching. Adding a variety of movements while engaged in a "thinking" game increases brain power.

Students think of the games in the classroom as fun and don't always realize they are learning in the process. By increasing movement, students mentally focus on the game and also build cognitive memory of the curriculum.

This resource is comprised of games to be played in a classroom that reinforce the current curriculum. For instance, the Student Tic-Tac-Toe game allows students to review while playing tic-tac-toe with their bodies. The teams think the objective is to get the first tic-tac-toe, but the real objective is to review information.

These activities will make learning easier, less stressful and more fun. Students will increase their concentration and have better retention as well as greater enjoyment and motivation.

No additional research or preparation is necessary for these games since you will use materials that the students are currently working on. Each activity is presented in the same format, so you can see at a glance what the objective of the game is, the preparation and materials needed and the directions for playing the game.

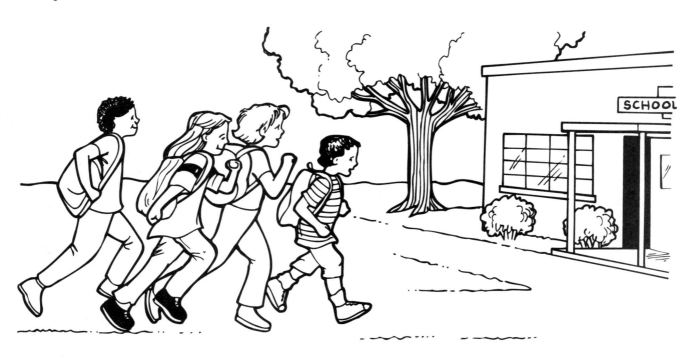

TLC10560 Copyright © Teaching & Learning Company, Carthage, IL 62321-0010

Knowledge Ball

Object of the Game

Review information from math, social studies, science, literature or reading lessons.

Preparation

Organize curriculum questions

Materials

a soft ball to toss

Directions

Have students make a circle around the room. Provide a topic for the game. Give one student a soft ball, like a tennis ball or beanbag. The student should throw the ball underhand to another student in the circle.

The student who catches the ball has five seconds to give one fact about the selected topic. If a student is unable to make a statement, he or she is out of the game. As students exit the game, they must sit quietly and watch the rest of the game in the center of the circle. Play until only one person is left.

For example, you are going to play the game using a book you are reading as a class:
The first student tosses the ball.
The second student catches the ball and states, "Johnny had straight black hair." He then tosses the ball to another student.
This student states, "The car wouldn't start so Johnny had to walk." Then she tosses the ball to someone else.
The next student catches the ball but cannot think of a comment. He is out of the game and must sit quietly in the center until everyone is eliminated but the winner.

An incentive (see incentive section) can be given to the winner.

Other Suggestions

a. Famous people (The first student names a famous person. The second must name what that person is famous for.)

b. Manners/Politeness (Each student must name a rule.)

c. Naming trees, flowers, birds, wild animals or domestic animals.

d. Life skills and how to show them.

Game Variations

a. Divide the class in half. Have sides face each other. Toss a volleyball or basketball back and forth down the line. Each student must state a fact when catching the ball or he or she is out.

b. As a student catches the ball, he or she must throw the ball in the air and state a fact before catching it. If correct, he or she tosses the ball to another student.

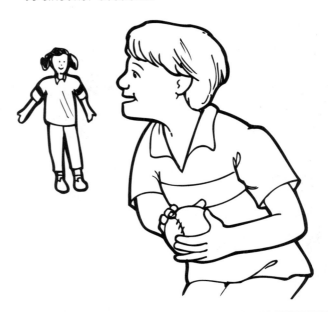

Knowledge Ball

Curriculum Variations

Geography

a. Capitals of U.S. (The first student names a state. The second student names the state's capital.)

b. Countries (The first student names a country. The second student names the continent where that country is located.)

c. Mountains (Each student must name a mountain range or individual mountain.)

Math

a. Multiplication tables (The first student tosses the ball and says "7." The second student tosses the ball and says "8." The third student must say "56.")

b. Counting in multiples (Be sure to provide a maximum.) Start a new counting sequence when someone misses or the maximum is reached.

c. Division (The first student gives a division problem like "56 divided by 8." The second student must give an answer and then state another problem before tossing the ball.)

Reading

a. Character analysis (Johnny's hair was red, Cynthia was bashful, etc.)

b. Settings (in Lake County, by Lake Annie, in the kitchen, etc.)

c. Plot (Johnny was afraid to fail; Marina knew the secret, etc.)

d. Sequencing (One person says a plot fact, and the person catching the ball states the next element of the plot.)

Science

a. Definitions

b. Chemical symbols (The first student states a chemical "gold." The second student must state the symbol "Au.")

Spelling

a. Give a word. The student catching the ball must spell the word correctly.

b. Syllables (Student must state how many syllables are in the spelling word.)

c. Definitions (Student must give the correct definition of the word.)

d. Synonyms/Antonyms

e. Sentences (Student must use the spelling word in a sentence.)

Vocabulary

a. Definitions (The first student gives a vocabulary word. The next student must give the definition.)

b. Synonyms/Antonyms (One student must give a word. The next student gives a word that means the same or the opposite.)

c. Sentences (One student says a vocabulary word. The next student uses that word in a sentence.)

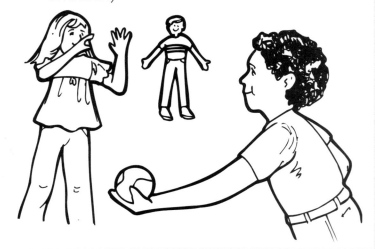

TLC10560 Copyright © Teaching & Learning Company, Carthage, IL 62321-0010

Word Chase

Object of the Game

Learn new words (or spelling words) and their definitions.

Preparation

Organize curriculum questions

Materials

dictionary or thesaurus per team

Directions

Separate the class into teams of four or five students. Give each team a dictionary or a textbook.

Have one student from each team come to you at a central location.

Give them all the same word.

Students then hurry back to their team and teams race to look up the word's definition.

When a team finds the word, they yell "got it!" The other teams must freeze.

The team that found the word reads the definition.

If the team is wrong, they're out. The remainder of the teams continue looking for the word.

Keep a score tallied on the board.

An incentive can be given to the winning team.

Game Variations

a. If enough dictionaries are available, make two-person teams. You can call out the word from the dictionary or textbook.

b. Synonym or antonym: Look for a word in a thesaurus and tells the teams, "I want a synonym for _____ that starts with the letter __." Students can find the answer by looking up the word and scanning the synonyms.

c. True and false questions: Give a word and a synonym for this word. The students should look up the word in the thesaurus and check if the word is really a synonym of the original word or not. The first team to find the answer calls out and the other teams freeze until it is determined if they are correct or not. (It is important to use the same thesaurus as the students.)

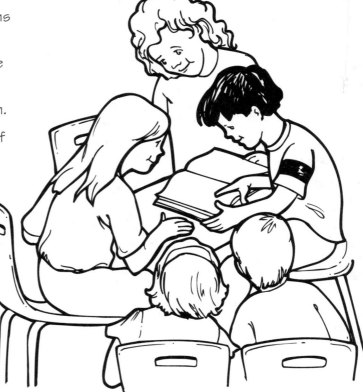

Eraser Tag

Object of the Game

Practice concepts while having fun.

Preparation

None

Materials

two clean erasers

Directions

On the board, have a student write a problem and then write another student's name. The student then places an eraser on his or her head and should wait in a designated area.

The student whose name is on the board must come and write the correct answer. The class yells "right!" or "wrong!" That student also places an eraser on his or her head and tries to tag the first student before 10 seconds are up.

Rules

a. Neither student may use their hands to hold the eraser on their head. If the eraser falls off, the student must stand still until the eraser is replaced.

b. The chaser only has 10 seconds to catch the first student.

c. If the chaser does tag the first student, that student gets to write a problem and another student's name on the board.

d. If the tag is not made within 10 seconds, the first student goes again.

Curriculum Variations

Geography

The first student writes the name of a continent on the board. The second student writes a country, city, river, mountain range or desert from that continent.

Grammar

Make plurals, possessives or plural possessives with singular nouns.

Math

Practice multiplication tables with this game.

Reading

Describe a character from a book. The second student must name the character.

Science

Chemical symbols—The first student writes a chemical on the board. (Example: gold). The second student must write the symbol (Example: Au).

Spelling

The first student writes a spelling word. Second student writes T (true) or F (false) behind the word to state if the word is spelled correctly or not. Since the class is the judge, this is a great way to review spelling words.

Game Variations

a. Separate the class into teams.

b. Students can hold something in their hands (like a ball on a spoon) instead of putting erasers on their heads.

No incentive is necessary for this game.

TLC10560 Copyright © Teaching & Learning Company, Carthage, IL 62321-0010

I Thought I Saw a Purple Cow

Object of the Game

Build unity in the class with the game. It is most effective when played at the beginning of the year to help students get to know each other.

Preparation

None

Materials

None

Directions

Select one student to sit in the "it" chair, facing away from the class.

Silently select another student.

This student recites, "I thought I saw a purple cow," or another selected nonsense sentence. This student should use a disguised voice.

The "it" student must guess who the speaker is. If the student is correct, he or she gets an incentive or a point, and is "it" again.

If the guess is incorrect, the speaker is the new "it" person.

Other nonsense statements are:
"I saw the cow jump over the moon."
"Julius Caesar has come to town."
"I sprayed a rainbow into the sky."

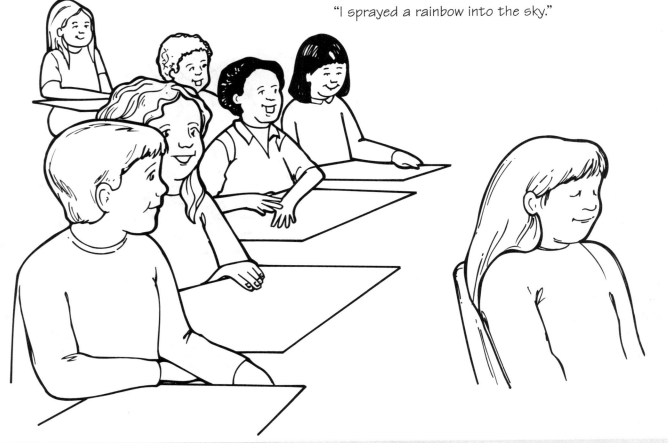

Question Quest

Object of the Game

Review curriculum topics by writing good questions.

Preparation

None

Materials

textbooks, paper, pencils

Directions

Separate the class into teams of four or five students each.

Give the teams 10 minutes to write at least five questions about the topic. Their chances of winning increase with the number of questions they have. The questions must be written down to count.

To start, give each team a number.

Team 1 begins by asking Team 2 a question.

Team 2 has one minute to answer. If they give the correct answer, they receive one point.

If they do not answer the question correctly, Team 3 gets a chance.

The question moves through the teams until a team answers correctly.

If no team answers correctly, Team 1 gets a point.

Then Team 2 asks Team 3 a question. Be sure to always go in numerical order so every team has an equal chance at points.

If a team runs out of questions, they are out of the game. They are not allowed to answer any more questions for points.
- One point for answering a question correctly.
- One point if no other team can answer their question.

The team with the most points at the end of the game can receive an incentive.

Curriculum Variations

Math

- Review long division or double-digit multiplication problems.
- Practice multiplication with decimals or fractions.
- Solve word problems involving sums of money or time.

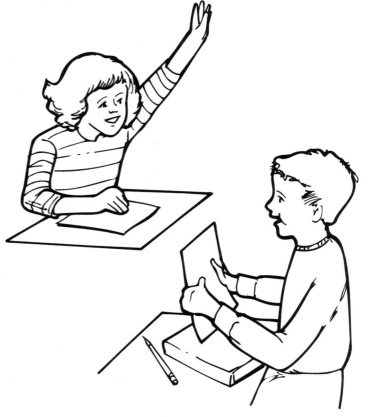

TLC10560 Copyright © Teaching & Learning Company, Carthage, IL 62321-0010

Impromptu Review

Object of the Game

Review information to help with test preparation.

Preparation

Write questions beforehand on single strips of paper and place in a bowl or hat. Write the names of all the students on other strips of paper and place in a separate bowl.

Materials

strips of paper, two bowls

Directions

Draw one name and one question. The student whose name is drawn stands up and answers the question. One point is given for a correct answer. Then draw another name and question. Encourage students to take notes because some of this information will be on the test. The notes will make a good study guide.

Game Variations

a. Have each student write one question related to the topic. Use these questions for the review.

b. When a student answers the question correctly, he or she then draws the next name and question.

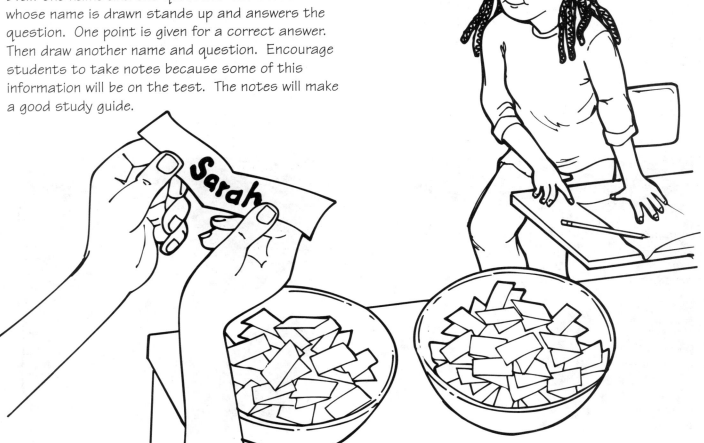

Math Whizzer

Object of the Game

Review addition, subtraction, multiplication and division.

Preparation

None

Materials

math problems, chalk, chalkboard

Directions

Separate the class into three to four teams. One member of each team should stand at the chalkboard. Call out a problem. Students must write the problem on the board and solve it. The first student to solve the problem says, "Done!" If the student is correct, that team gets one point. If the student is incorrect, the others have additional time to solve the problem. The first team with the correct answer gets a point.

Rules

a. Every member of a team must take a turn.

b. Only one point is earned for each correct answer.

c. If a member of the team helps the member at the board, then that team is disqualified for the round.

Game Variations

a. Divide the class in half. If one team gives the incorrect answer, then the other team has as much time as they need to get it right.

b. Allow all members of the team to help with the problem. Remind them that when they call out an answer, the other teams can hear it too.

c. After the students write the problem on the chalkboard, they go back to their teams to figure out the answer. They must return to the chalkboard and write the solution before yelling "done!"

The winners can be given an incentive.

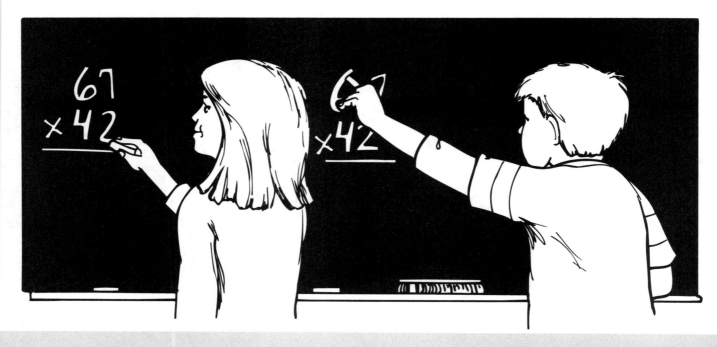

TLC10560 Copyright © Teaching & Learning Company, Carthage, IL 62321-0010

Poetry in Motion

Object of the Game

Teach students rhyme and rhyme patterns as well as teamwork.

Preparation

Create a list of words students can use to rhyme.

Materials

paper, pencils

Directions

Divide the class into teams, with four or five students on each team. Read a word and have the teams list four words that rhyme with that word. After listing the four additional words, each team should write a quick verse using all five rhyming words. At the end of five minutes, each team reads their verse out loud. Have the class vote on the best poem.

Rules

a. Give five minutes for each word used in this exercise.

b. The verse must rhyme.

c. All five of the words must be used.

Game Variations

Give three spelling words. Each team has two minutes to write the three words in a sentence. When the sentences are read, the best one receives a point.

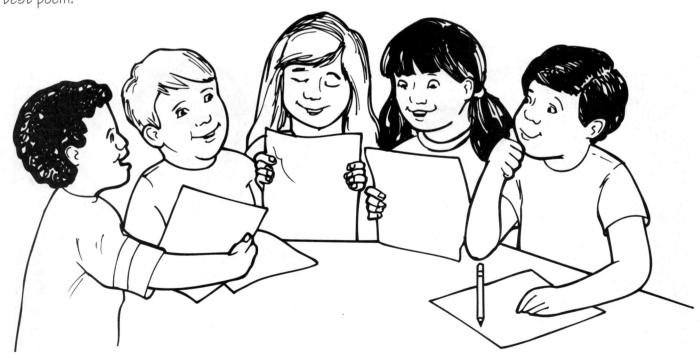

TLC10560 Copyright © Teaching & Learning Company, Carthage, IL 62321-0010

Spell-a-Round

Object of the Game

Help students concentrate and think fast. It also helps get a class motivated first thing in the morning.

Preparation

None

Materials

one number for each student, a bowl

Directions

Place one number for each student in a bowl. Have students draw a number. Start the round by giving a word and spelling it correctly. The student with number one gives a new word that starts with the last letter of the previous word and spells it correctly. The student with number two gives a new word starting with the last letter of the word from student one. Go around the room three times.

Rules

The student must spell the word correctly. If the word is spelled incorrectly, the student is eliminated.

The student has 10 seconds to think of a word. If the student cannot think of a word, he or she is eliminated. Trying to eliminate other students is part of the game.

Points

• One point is given for each letter in the word the student spells. The longer the word, the more points a student receives.

• An extra point is awarded if the word is/was one of the class spelling words.

After three rounds, the student with the most points can receive an incentive.

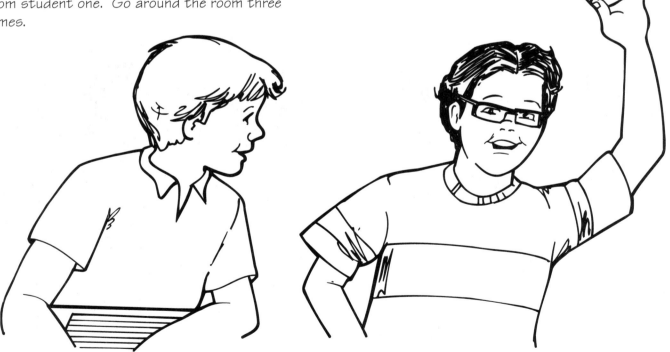

TLC10560 Copyright © Teaching & Learning Company, Carthage, IL 62321-0010

Match-Catch

Object of the Game

Help students memorize information from subjects they are currently studying.

Preparation

Questions or a list of words

Materials

None

Directions

Divide the class in half. Have the teams stand facing each other in two long lines.

The first person in line makes a statement that needs a match. (Example: Ruler of England)

The first student on the other team must answer correctly (Example match: King George III) or is eliminated. If the student cannot find a match, then the first student has "caught" the second student. If the student answers correctly, then he or she makes a statement to try and catch the next person on the other team. The student who asked the question goes to the end of the line. The play follows down the line, moving students up as others are eliminated. The last person standing is the winner.

Rules

The student trying to "catch," must know an answer to their statement. All answers must come from memory. No notes allowed.

Curriculum Variations

Grammar

The first student says a sentence that might or might not be grammatically correct. The second student must either state "The sentence is correct" or correct the grammatical error.

Spelling

The first student gives a word. The second student must spell it correctly or give its definition.

Game Variations

The class stands in a circle with the teacher in the middle. The teacher gives the statement and students take turns answering. If they cannot find a match, they are eliminated.

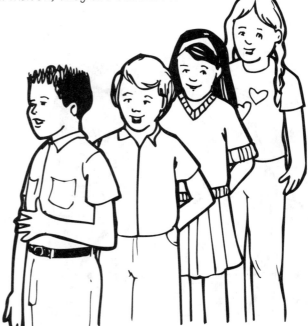

TLC10560 Copyright © Teaching & Learning Company, Carthage, IL 62321-0010

Student Tic-Tac-Toe

Object of the Game

Review and practice information.

Preparation

Curriculum questions, cards with Xs and Os

Materials

nine chairs set in three rows, three chairs per row (like tic-tac-toe)

Directions

Divide the class in half. Give half the students cards with a large O on them. The other students should get cards with a large X on them. (8½" x 11" pages with a large X or O written on them and a string attached long enough to be placed around their necks works well.)

Students should line up with the Os on one side of the chairs and the Xs on the other. Ask the first student a question. If the student answers correctly, he or she picks a seat in the tic-tac-toe chairs. If the student answers incorrectly, he or she goes to the end of the line and the other team gets a turn. Play continues until one team makes a tic-tac-toe. Award one point for tic-tac-toe.

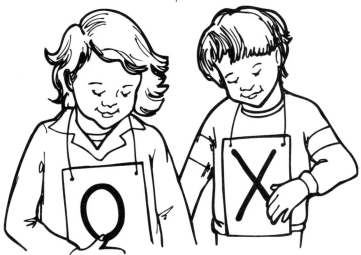

Rules

When the question is asked, only one student may answer. If another student helps with the answer, both are eliminated and the other team gets the next question.

Students sitting in the chairs must keep their cards in front of them so the student trying to find a place in the tic-tac-toe chairs can see where to sit. The other students cannot help make the choice.

The team with the most points at the end of the game can receive an incentive.

Curriculum Variations

Health

Review parts of the body or diseases.

Math

Any form of math question may be asked, including multiplication tables, math terminology, fractions, double-digit addition or subtraction by memory.

Science

Practice chemical symbols or current topics.

Social Studies

Ask questions about current studies.

Spelling

Practice new and old spelling words.

Mix

Have a variety of questions to include all subjects.

TLC10560 Copyright © Teaching & Learning Company, Carthage, IL 62321-0010

Social Studies Scramble

Object of the Game

Review content in social studies or other textbooks.

Preparation

Topics or questions from textbook

Materials

textbook, pencils, paper, overhead projector

Directions

Cut two pieces of paper into one-inch squares.

Prepare questions from the current chapter in the social studies textbook. Then write one question at a time on the overhead projector. When finished, call "Go!" and show the question.

The students should race to find the answer in their textbook. When someone finds the answer, he or she yells, "Got it!"

Call "Stop!" and have students tell where the answer is found (page and paragraph). If correct, give the student one square of construction paper. Other students should read and take notes on the answer.

Play continues until all the questions are asked. The top five (or ten) students can receive an incentive.

Curriculum Variations

Dictionary Practice

Give a vocabulary word from current social studies unit. Students must find and read the definition.

Literature

Use to review the current reading book.

Game Variations

Divide the class into teams. Have two social studies books and dictionaries on a desk at the front of the room. When the question is uncovered, one student from each team races to find the answer.

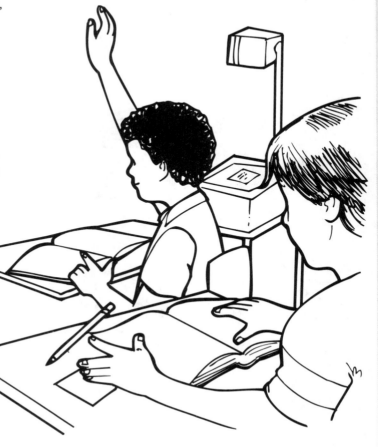

Mystery Can Game

Object of the Game

Develop deductive thinking skills. Also practice teamwork and build community.

Preparation

None

Materials

one 32-ounce coffee can, decorated

Directions

Choose one student to take the mystery can home and place an object inside. The next day, place the can at the front of the classroom with the lid closed. The rest of the students ask questions that can be answered with "yes" or "no." Each student can ask two questions. The first student to figure out what is inside the can wins. Then select a new student to take the mystery can home.

Rules

No student is allowed to look inside or pick up the can.

Game Variations

a. After telling the class if the contents are animal, vegetable or mineral, the student allows 20 questions before giving a clue to the can's contents.

b. The can may go home with a different student each night and whatever is placed in the can must follow a theme for the entire week. (colors, toys, sports, food, etc.)

c. The student must place something in the can that relates to a current unit of study in the classroom.

d. The student gives three clues. Each student who wishes to guess writes an answer on a piece of paper. The student who brought the can reads the written responses and determines a winner.

e. Instead of the teacher giving an incentive, the student who took the can home may be responsible for the prize given by bringing it himself.

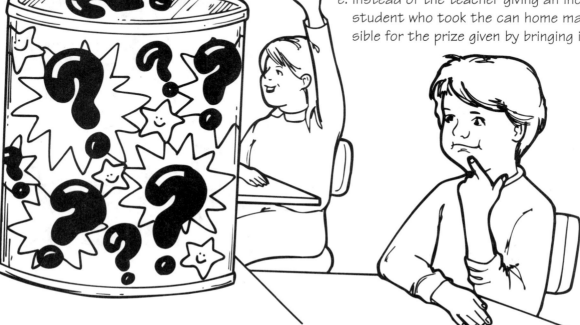

TLC10560 Copyright © Teaching & Learning Company, Carthage, IL 62321-0010

Definition Search

Object of the Game

Learn uncommon or unique words and their meanings.

Preparation

Copies of words and definitions, cut apart

Materials

None

Directions

Copy page 20 and cut the words and definitions apart. There will be 16 words and 16 definitions. Distribute one word or definition to each student.

To play the game, have one student call out a word. If another student thinks he has the definition to that word, he raises his hand and gives the definition. If the student is correct, he gets one point and the word holder is out of the game. If the student is wrong, the word holder receives a point and reads the word on a subsequent turn.

Students holding definitions may only try three times to find the correct word for their definitions. If they are not correct after three tries, they are out of the game.

You can write the points on the board or hand out pieces of construction paper, paper clips, etc. Extra points can be awarded at the end of the game to a student who can recite a word and its definition (not that student's word or definition).

Note: These words are "old-fashioned" words that were used in the 1800s or early 1900s and are no longer used. Discuss other little-used words or have students ask their parents for words they remember from their youth that are no longer used.

Answers for Teacher

spider: A cast iron pan with a handle used for frying food

wrapper: A loose outer garment; an article of dress fitted loosely around a person

cambric: Cotton or linen cloth, printed with flowers and other patterns in a number of different colors

chintz: A cotton cloth with a printed pattern, usually glazed, used for curtains

arnica: The roots of an herb used in the form of a lotion for bruises or sprains

jake staff: Used for supporting a compass

butteris: A steel instrument for paring the hooves of horses

leg-of-mutton: A puffy sleeve from the shoulder to the elbow

jabot: A trimming of a piece of lace usually ruffled. Worn by women down the front of their dresses

leghorn: A plaiting used for hats and bonnets made from straw, cut green and bleached

gimp: A narrow ornamental fabric of silk, wool or cotton, used as trimming for dresses, furniture, etc.

chambray: A lightweight clothing fabric with white filling yarns

butterine: An artificial spread of margarine

gem: A muffin made with coarse flour

shivaree: A serenade played for a newly married couple, using pots and pans and horns

Tin Lizzie: A nickname for the Model T Ford automobile; a small, inexpensive early automobile

Definition Search

spider	A lightweight clothing fabric with white filling yarns
wrapper	A plaiting used for hats and bonnets made from straw, cut green and bleached
cambric	A steel instrument for paring the hooves of horses
chintz	A cast iron pan with a handle used for frying food
arnica	A muffin made with coarse flour
jake staff	A trimming of a piece of lace, usually ruffled. Worn by women down the front of their dresses
butteris	A cotton cloth with a printed pattern, usually glazed, used for curtains
leg-of-mutton	A puffy sleeve from the shoulder to the elbow
jabot	A serenade played for a newly married couple, using pots and pans and horns
leghorn	An artificial spread of margarine
gimp	Cotton or linen cloth, printed with flowers and other patterns in a number of different colors
chambray	A loose outer garment; an article of dress fitted loosely around a person
butterine	The roots of an herb used in the form of a lotion for bruises or sprains
gem	A narrow ornamental fabric (silk, wool or cotton) used as trim on dresses, furniture, etc.
shivaree	Used for supporting a compass
Tin Lizzie	A nickname for the Model T Ford automobile; a small, inexpensive early automobile

TLC10560 Copyright © Teaching & Learning Company, Carthage, IL 62321-0010

Spelling Baseball

Object of the Game

Review spelling words.

Preparation

Copy playing cards on page 22, cut apart and place in a bowl.

Materials

list of spelling words, heavy paper, bowl

Directions

Divide the class in half. Tape a home plate and first, second and third bases around the room in a baseball diamond shape. Team 1 is "up to bat," and Team 2 is "out in the field." The "pitcher" reads a spelling word, the student at bat must spell the word correctly. If correct, the student draws a card from the bowl. After reading the card, place it back in the bowl.

The second student from Team 1 is now at bat. The pitcher reads another spelling word. Every student who spells correctly draws a card. An incorrect spelling is an out. Three outs and the other team is up to bat.

If a student makes it to home plate, a run is scored. The team with the most runs wins the game.

Game Variations

Use to review other curriculum topics. The pitcher can pitch a question and the batter must answer it correctly.

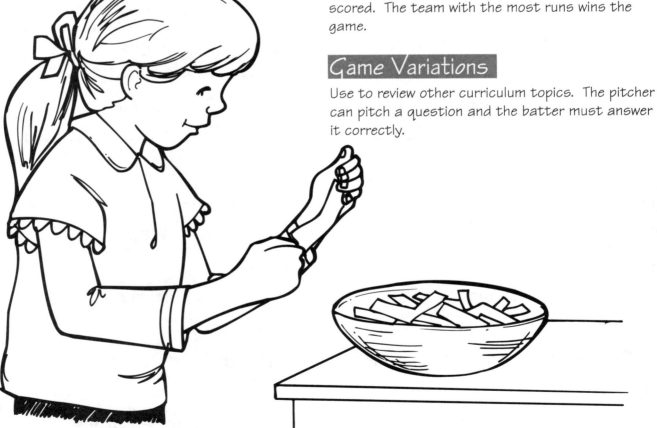

Spelling Baseball

Out at first	Out at first
Out at first	Out at first
Reached first on an error	Reached first on an error
Base hit	Base hit
Base hit	Base hit
Catcher touches bat	Triple
Home run	Double
Double	Double
Walk	Walk
Triple	Triple
Pitcher hits batter with ball	Pitcher hits batter with ball
Fielder's choice	Fielder's choice

TLC10560 Copyright © Teaching & Learning Company, Carthage, IL 62321-0010

Memory Challenge

Object of the Game

Build memory skills and learn more about class-mates.

Preparation

None

Materials

None

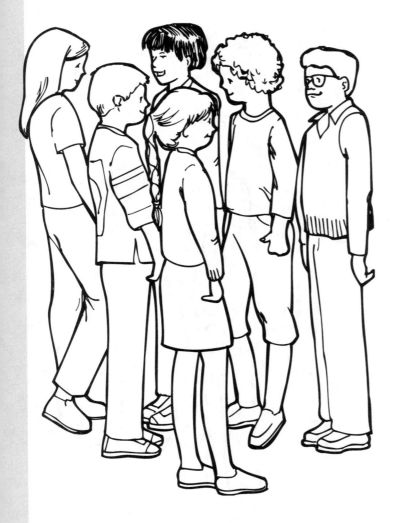

Directions

One half of the class forms a circle, shoulder to shoulder with arms at their sides, facing out.

The other half of the class forms a circle outside that circle, facing in.

Each student in the outside circle tells the student in the inside circle something about his or her summer or vacation. After 10 seconds, the inside circle rotates clockwise one student. The student tells the current partner something different, and the circle moves again. This continues until the circles are again back to the original set of partners.

The inside students recite what they remember about each outside student. The winner is the student who remembers the most information.

Then have circles switch places and repeat.

There are two winners—one for each circle.

Curriculum Variations

Can also be used to review current curriculum topics.

Making Time

Object of the Game

Review curriculum content.

Preparation

Curriculum questions, two 8½" x 11" papers with the number 12 written on them

Materials

paper, tape

Directions

Tape a sheet with "12" to the floor in two different locations. Have students form two circles (12 students each). One student should stand on each of the 12s. Explain to them that they are creating the face of the clock. They must remember who started the game standing on the 12.

Read a question to the first clock group. The student standing on the 12 answers the question. If correct, the circle moves ahead one hour. If incorrect, the students may not move. Then ask the next clock group a question, reminding the students to pay attention because some questions may be repeated.

Continue until one of the clocks returns to its original position. That team wins.

Questions can come from any curriculum topic.

An incentive can be given to the students in the winning clock group.

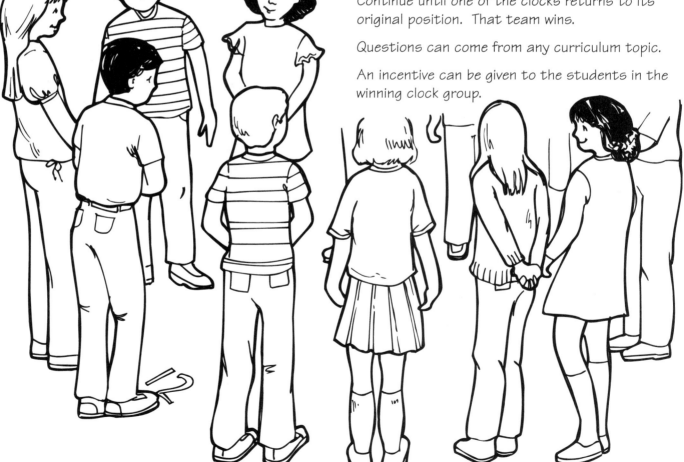

TLC10560 Copyright © Teaching & Learning Company, Carthage, IL 62321-0010

Race to the Captain

Object of the Game

Review curriculum topics.

Preparation

List of curriculum questions

Materials

None

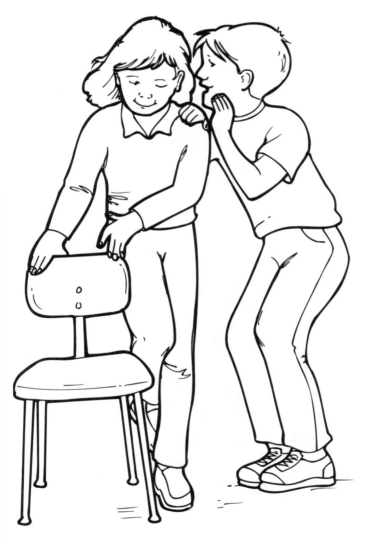

Directions

Divide the class in half. Each team selects a captain. The captains should sit the same distance from their teams, and the two captains should not sit close together.

Ask a question. Any team member who knows the answer must rush to tell the captain. The first captain to stand up is allowed to give the answer.

If the question is answered correctly, the team receives two points. If the question is answered incorrectly, the other team has a chance to answer. If they answer correctly, they receive one point.

The team with the most points receives an incentive.

Game Variations

If the question is answered correctly, the captain must shoot a ball or a beanbag at a container (like a garbage can). The containers must be placed an equal distance from the captains.

An incentive is given to the team that makes the most baskets.

"Old Maid" Game

Object of the Game

Review curriculum topics.

Preparation

List of questions

Materials

an object for each student with his or her name on it

Directions

Give each student an object like a beanbag, a chip or a piece of cardboard with his or her name on it. Ask a question and allow the first student who raises a hand to answer it.

If the answer is correct, the object goes into a hat or box. This student may not answer any more questions. Only students with an object may answer.

If the answer is incorrect, the student must hold on to the object and cannot answer another question until only 10 students are left. They may then get into the game again.

The last student holding an object is the Old Maid and loses the game.

Curriculum Variations

Math

Use multiplication problems, thought problems, addition or subtraction problems.

Reading

Ask questions from the current reading or social studies book.

Spelling

Practice new and old spelling words.

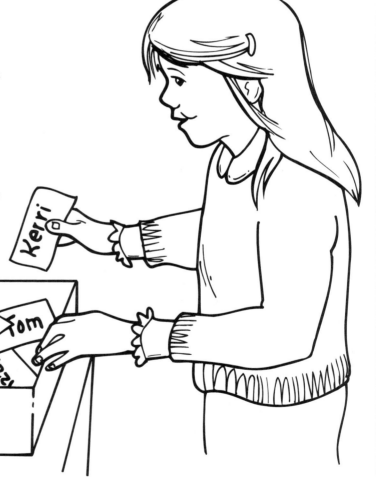

TLC10560 Copyright © Teaching & Learning Company, Carthage, IL 62321-0010

The Presidents Game

Object of the Game

Teaches about the U.S. Presidents, but can be used for any other curriculum content by making new cards.

Preparation

Make one copy each of the question pages (pages 30-32) and one copy of the Presidents' names (pages 33-34). Cut the names apart and place in a bowl.

Materials

questions and Presidents' name cards, bowl, tape

Directions

Each student draws from the bowl, receiving a question or a President's name and pins it to his or her shirt. Taking turns, the students who have drawn the Presidents' names walk around the students wearing the questions, trying to find the correct fit with their given President. If a student finds the correct question to fit his or her President, he or she receives one point. Both students move out of the game.

After this round, the students with questions take turns walking around the students with Presidents' names trying to find the correct Presidents for their questions.

Play continues until all Presidents and questions are matched up. The names and questions then go back into the bowl.

The teacher should warn students to listen for correct as well as incorrect answers because the game will be replayed many times until all students are familiar with which question belongs with which President.

An incentive could be given to the first student who is able to match a President with a question or to all who match up correctly.

EXTRA CREDIT: On pages 35-36 are more questions about Presidents that can be given to the whole class or placed on strips and handed out when the first set of questions have been used several times.

Game Variations

a. Write the Presidents' names on the board. Number the questions on the copied pages and have students write the number of the question he or she believes is correct behind each President's name. The teacher states which ones are correct but still erases them when it is the next student's turn. The new students coming to the board must remember which ones are correct and which ones are incorrect.

b. Pass out the cards randomly to students with equal questions and names.

The Presidents Game

Answers to President Questions (pages 30-32)

1. Who is the only President buried in Washington, D.C.? *Woodrow Wilson*
2. Who was the only President to serve as Speaker of the House? *James Polk*
3. Who was the only President to serve two nonconsecutive terms? *Grover Cleveland*
4. Who was the first President to be sworn into office on an airplane? *Lyndon B. Johnson*
5. Who was the only man to serve as both President and Chief Justice of the Supreme Court? *William Taft*
6. Which President lived the shortest time? *John F. Kennedy (46 years old)*
7. Who was the first President to live in the White House? *John Adams*
8. Which President had 15 children? *John Tyler*
9. Who was the first President to be inaugurated in Washington, D.C.? *Thomas Jefferson*
10. Which President served the shortest time in office? *William H. Harrison (In 1841—one month)*
11. Which President ran for office without an opponent? *James Monroe*
12. Which President never married? *James Buchanan*
13. Which President issued the Proclamation of Emancipation? *Abraham Lincoln*
14. Which President lost his 11-year-old son in a train wreck just before becoming President and lost his wife to illness during his presidency? *Franklin Pierce*
15. Which President's picture is on the one dollar bill? *George Washington*
16. Which President's picture is on a dime? *Franklin D. Roosevelt*
17. Who was President when the Soviet Union broke into individual states and the Communist party lost control? *George H. Bush*
18. Who was the first President to have his term of office limited by the Constitution? *Dwight D. Eisenhower*
19. Which President's picture is on the fifty dollar bill? *Ulysses S. Grant*
20. Which President's campaign speech stated, "A chicken in every pot and a car in every garage"? *Herbert Hoover*
21. Which President won the Nobel Peace Prize for helping organize a peace treaty between Egypt and Israel? *James Carter*
22. Who was President when terrorists attacked the twin towers of the World Trade Center in New York on September 11, 2001? *George W. Bush*
23. Which President ordered the atom bomb attacks on Hiroshima and Nagasaki, Japan? *Harry S. Truman*
24. Which President lived in the White House when it was burned by the British? *James Madison*
25. Who was President when the Wright Brothers made their first airplane flight? *Theodore Roosevelt*
26. Which President's picture is on the twenty dollar bill? *Andrew Jackson*
27. Which President was elected over his opponent by only one electoral vote? *Rutherford B. Hayes*
28. Who was the only man to serve as Vice President and President who did not win an election to either office? *Gerald R. Ford*
29. Who was President during the Klondike Gold Rush? *William McKinley*
30. Which President starred in over 50 films before seeking the presidency? *Ronald Reagan*
31. Which President was part of "Watergate," the biggest government scandal in U.S. history? *Richard Nixon*
32. Who was considered the weakest President in U.S. history because he was weak-willed and a poor judge of character? *Warren G. Harding*
33. Which President appointed more women and minority members to his cabinet than any previous President? *William Clinton*
34. Who was President when the first postage stamp came into use? *Martin Van Buren*
35. Who was President when the first flight over the North Pole took place? *Calvin Coolidge*
36. Which President saw the Brooklyn Bridge completed in 1883? *Chester A. Arthur*
37. Which President, before leaving office, pardoned all Southerners who had taken part in the Civil War? *Andrew Johnson*
38. Who was President when the first overland mail service by wagon served America? *Zachary Taylor (1850—It took 30 days to travel from Independence, Missouri, to Salt Lake City, Utah)*
39. Which President helped pass the law requiring children to go to school? *Millard Fillmore (In Massachusetts, 1852)*
40. Who was President when Daniel Webster's dictionary was published? *John Quincy Adams*
41. Who was the last President to be born in a log cabin? *James A. Garfield*

TLC10560 Copyright © Teaching & Learning Company, Carthage, IL 62321-0010

The Presidents Game

Extra Credit Questions Answers (page 35)

1. Who was the first President sworn into office by a woman? *Lyndon B. Johnson by Judge Sarah T. Hughes*

2. Which Presidents signed the Constitution? *George Washington and James Madison*

3. Which Presidents died on the Fourth of July? *Thomas Jefferson (1826), John Adams (1826), James Monroe (1831)*

4. Which Presidents were assassinated? *Abraham Lincoln, James A. Garfield, William McKinley, John F. Kennedy*

5. Who was the first President to speak on the radio? *Woodrow Wilson*

6. Who were the only two Presidents to be sworn into office by a former President? *Calvin Coolidge and Herbert Hoover (by Taft)*

7. Who was the first President nominated by a national political convention? *Andrew Jackson*

8. Who was President when the U.S. Forest Service was established? *Theodore Roosevelt*

9. Who was President when the Social Security Act was passed by Congress? *Franklin D. Roosevelt*

10. Who was the first President to speak on television? *Franklin D. Roosevelt*

11. Who was President when the U.S. flag obtained its 50 stars? *Dwight D. Eisenhower*

12. Which President established the Peace Corps? *John F. Kennedy*

13. Who was President when man flew in space for the first time? *John F. Kennedy*

14. Which President worked on a peanut farm when he was a boy? *James Carter*

15. What President said, "A house divided against itself cannot stand"? *Abraham Lincoln*

16. Which President saw the Hubble Space Telescope launched into orbit? *George H. Bush*

17. Who was President when the U.S. Marine Corps and the Dept. of the Navy were established? *John Adams*

18. Who was President when Amendment 16 was passed giving Congress authority to levy a national income tax on the citizens of the U.S.? *William Taft*

19. Who was the only grandson of a President who also became President? *Benjamin Harrison*

20. Which President received a smaller number of popular votes than his opponent but received more votes from the Electoral College to become President? *George W. Bush*

21. Who was the first President to travel in a jet plane? *Dwight D. Eisenhower*

22. Who was President when the first part of the International Space Station was launched? *William Clinton (1998 with more than 15 nations involved)*

23. Who was the first President to visit a foreign country while in office? *Theodore Roosevelt*

24. Who was President when the Unknown Soldier was buried at Arlington National Cemetery? *Warren G. Harding*

25. Which President created the Department of the Interior on his last day as President? *James Polk*

26. Who was governor of Texas before becoming President? *George W. Bush*

27. Which President increased the respect for the U.S. flag ordering the flag be flown over all government buildings and every school? *Benjamin Harrison*

28. Who was President when the first woman lawyer practiced before the Supreme Court? *Rutherford B. Hayes (Belva Ann Lockwood, 1879)*

29. Who was President when the 26th Amendment lowered the voting age to 18 years old? *Richard Nixon*

30. Which President talked to Neil Armstrong and Buzz Aldrin when they walked on the moon? *Richard Nixon (Apollo 11, July 20, 1969)*

31. Who was President when the government moved from Philadelphia to Washington, D.C.? *John Adams*

32. Who was President when Alaska was purchased from Russia in 1867? *Andrew Johnson*

33. Who was President when the Confederate States of America was formed? *James Buchanan*

34. Who was President when the United Nations was established? *Harry S. Truman*

35. Who was the only President to be acquitted when Congress tried to impeach him? *Andrew Johnson*

The Presidents Game
Questions

1. Who is the only President buried in Washington, D.C.?

2. Who was the only President to serve as Speaker of the House?

3. Who was the only President to serve two nonconsecutive terms?

4. Who was the first President to be sworn into office on an airplane?

5. Who was the only man to serve as both President and Chief Justice of the Supreme Court?

6. Which President lived the shortest time?

7. Who was the first President to live in the White House?

8. Which President had 15 children?

9. Who was the first President to be inaugurated in Washington, D.C.?

10. Which President served the shortest time in office?

11. Which President ran for office without an opponent?

12. Which President never married?

13. Which President issued the Proclamation of Emancipation?

14. Which President lost his 11-year-old son in a train wreck just before becoming President and lost his wife to illness during his presidency?

TLC10560 Copyright © Teaching & Learning Company, Carthage, IL 62321-0010

The Presidents Game Questions

15. Which President's picture is on the one dollar bill?

16. Which President's picture is on a dime?

17. Who was President when the Soviet Union broke into individual states and the Communist party lost control?

18. Who was the first President to have his term of office limited by the Constitution?

19. Which President's picture is on the fifty dollar bill?

20. Which President's campaign speech stated, "A chicken in every pot and a car in every garage"?

21. Which President won the Nobel Peace Prize for helping organize a peace treaty between Egypt and Israel?

22. Who was President when terrorists attacked the twin towers of the World Trade Center in New York on September 11, 2001?

23. Which President ordered the atom bomb attacks on Hiroshima and Nagasaki, Japan?

24. Which President lived in the White House when it was burned by the British?

25. Who was President when the Wright Brothers made their first airplane flight?

26. Which President's picture is on the twenty dollar bill?

27. Which President was elected over his opponent by only one electoral vote?

28. Who was the only man to serve as Vice President and President who did not win an election to either office?

The Presidents Game Questions

29. Who was President during the Klondike Gold Rush?

30. Which President starred in over 50 films before seeking the presidency?

31. Which President was part of "Watergate," the biggest government scandal in U.S. history?

32. Who was considered the weakest President in U.S. history
because he was weak-willed and a poor judge of character?

33. Which President appointed more women and minority members
to his cabinet than any previous President?

34. Who was President when the first postage stamp came into use?

35. Who was President when the first flight over the North Pole took place?

36. Which President saw the Brooklyn Bridge completed in 1883?

37. Which President, before leaving office,
pardoned all southerners who had taken part in the Civil War?

38. Who was President when the first overland mail service by wagon served America?

39. Which President helped pass the law requiring children to go to school?

40. Who was President when Daniel Webster's dictionary was published?

41. Who was the last President to be born in a log cabin?

TLC10560 Copyright © Teaching & Learning Company, Carthage, IL 62321-0010

The Presidents Game
Presidents' Names

Woodrow Wilson	James Polk
Grover Cleveland	John Adams
Lyndon B. Johnson	William Taft
James Buchanan	Theodore Roosevelt
John F. Kennedy	Andrew Jackson
John Tyler	Thomas Jefferson
Franklin D. Roosevelt	William H. Harrison
James Monroe	Dwight D. Eisenhower
Warren G. Harding	Ulysses S. Grant
Harry S. Truman	James Madison
George Washington	Abraham Lincoln

The Presidents Game
Presidents' Names

Franklin Pierce	Rutherford B. Hayes
Herbert Hoover	Calvin Coolidge
Ronald Reagan	William McKinley
James Carter	Zachary Taylor
Richard Nixon	Chester A. Arthur
James A. Garfield	John Quincy Adams
George W. Bush	Martin Van Buren
Gerald R. Ford	William Clinton
Millard Fillmore	Andrew Johnson
George H. Bush	

TLC10560 Copyright © Teaching & Learning Company, Carthage, IL 62321-0010

The Presidents Game
Extra Credit

Name_____

1. Who was the first President sworn into office by a woman? _____

2. Which Presidents signed the Constitution? _____

3. Which Presidents died on the Fourth of July?_____

_____

4. Which Presidents were assassinated? _____

_____

5. Who was the first President to speak on the radio? _____

6. Who were the only two Presidents to be sworn into office by a former President? _____

_____

7. Who was the first President nominated by a national political convention? _____

8. Who was President when the U.S. Forest Service was established? _____

9. Who was President when the Social Security Act was passed by Congress? _____

10. Who was the first President to speak on television? _____

11. Who was President when the U.S. flag obtained its 50 stars? _____

12. Which President established the Peace Corps?_____

13. Who was President when man flew in space for the first time? _____

14. Which President worked on a peanut farm when he was a boy? _____

15. What President said, "A house divided against itself cannot stand"? _____

16. Which President saw the Hubble Space Telescope launched into orbit?_____

17. Who was President when the U.S. Marine Corps and the Dept. of the Navy were established?

_____

18. Who was President when Amendment 16 was passed giving Congress authority to levy a national

income tax on the citizens of the U.S.? _____

19. Who was the only grandson of a President who also became President?_____

The Presidents Game
Extra Credit

Name_____

20. Which President received a smaller number of popular votes than his opponent but received more votes from the Electoral College to become President? _____

21. Who was the first President to travel in a jet plane? _____

22. Who was President when the first part of the International Space Station was launched?

_____

23. Who was the first President to visit a foreign country while in office? _____

24. Who was President when the Unknown Soldier was buried at Arlington National Cemetery?

_____

25. Which President created the Department of the Interior on his last day as President?

_____

26. Who was governor of Texas before becoming President? _____

27. Which President increased the respect for the U.S. flag ordering the flag be flown over all government buildings and every school? _____

28. Who was President when the first woman lawyer practiced before the Supreme Court?

_____

29. Who was President when the 26th Amendment lowered the voting age to 18 years old?_____

30. Which President talked to Neil Armstrong and Buzz Aldrin when they walked on the moon?

_____

31. Who was President when the government moved from Philadelphia to Washington D.C.?

_____

32. Who was President when Alaska was purchased from Russia in 1867?_____

33. Who was President when the Confederate States of America was formed? _____

34. Who was President when the United Nations was established?_____

35. Who was the only President to be acquitted when Congress tried to impeach him?_____

TLC10560 Copyright © Teaching & Learning Company, Carthage, IL 62321-0010

Classroom Short Story

Object of the Game

Practice writing short stories, creating characters and conflict, and describing a setting where the action takes place.

Preparation

None

Materials

a notebook, pencil

Directions

Choose a student to write the opening paragraph of a class story (average of 30 words). The student should leave the last sentence unfinished. The next student then reads the paragraph and writes the next one, leaving the last sentence unfinished. This continues until everyone in the class has a chance to write part of the story.

Younger children may only add a sentence instead of a paragraph.

Rules

1. Each paragraph should be approximately 30 words.
2. Allow one day for a student to read the story and complete a new paragraph.

Game Variations

a. Define the characters and the conflict, and write the first paragraph before giving to the students.

b. As a class, discuss who the characters will be and what the conflict is, then write the first paragraph together.

c. Have a contest to title the story.

d. Have the class illustrate the story and make a book.

e. Create the story as a class with each student stating one sentence. Tape the story to be played later.

Classroom Discussion

(After the story is finished)

• Did you understand the characters' motives and goal?

• How many characters were in the story?

• How old was the main character?

• How did the conflict change the story?

• Did the setting help you understand the conflict?

• Did the character solve the conflict?

• What was the genre of the story? (Science fiction? Romance? Adventure?)

• How long did the story last? (One day? Two years?)

• What could have enhanced the story?

• Did the story have a satisfying conclusion?

• What should the title be?

Ding Dong Bell

Object of the Game

Review basic math facts, like factors and multiples.

Preparation

None

Materials

None

Directions

Have the class form a circle around the room. Give each student a number starting with 1. The students should continue counting around the circle.

Round 1—Add a multiple.
If the multiple is 2, the student who is number "2" says "ding" instead. Every time a number is a multiple of 2 (2, 4, 6, 8, 10, etc.), the student must say "ding."

Round 2—Add a second multiple.
After one or two times around the circle, add a second multiple.

If you add multiples of 5, every time a number is a multiple of 5 (5, 10, 15, 20, etc.) the student must say "dong." When reaching a number like 10, the student must say "ding-dong" because 10 is a multiple of both 2 and 5.

Round 3—Add a third multiple.
After one or two times around the circle, add a third multiple, like the multiple of 3. Every time a number is a multiple of 3, the student must say "bell." For a number like 6, the student must say "ding-bell" because 6 is a multiple of both 2 and 3.

Rules

1. Students have five seconds to answer.
2. If a student misses, he or she is out of the game.
3. The game continues until only five students are left.

Give an incentive to the winners.

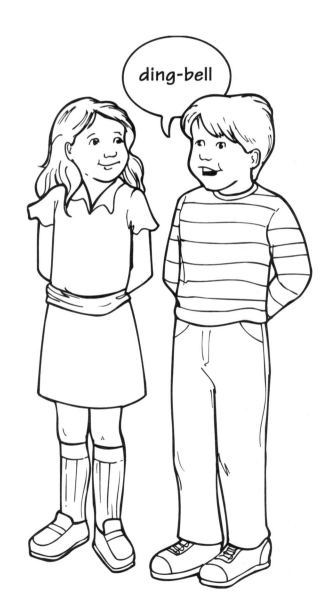

ding-bell

TLC10560 Copyright © Teaching & Learning Company, Carthage, IL 62321-0010

If/Then Game

Object of the Game

Review curriculum

Preparation

None

Materials

None

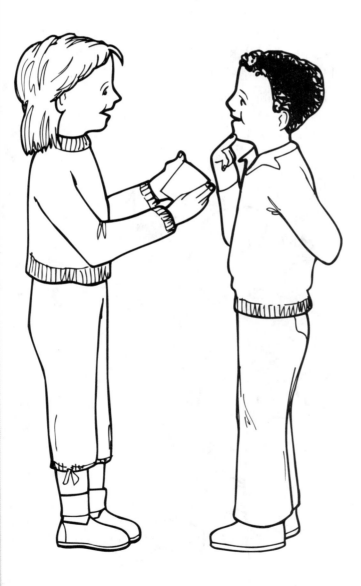

Directions

Give students time to prepare five "if/then" statements each. If/then statements can be about anything the students are currently studying.

Examples:

• True statement: "If *rhyming* is spelled R-H-Y-M-I-N-G, then George Washington was our first President."

• False statement: "If 3 x 12 = 34, then Alabama borders Kentucky.

After the students have written their questions, divide the class in half. The teams should form a line facing each other. Go down the line with the students asking each other their questions. The other team's student must answer "true" or "false." If the answer is false, the student must reword the statement to make it true.

If a student answers incorrectly, that student is out of the game. Continue the game until one team is completely eliminated. The other team is the winner.

Game Variations

You can write the questions and provide them to the students.

Musical Circles

Object of the Game

Review curriculum topics.

Preparation

List of spelling words or curriculum questions

Materials

pencil, paper, CDs and a CD player

Directions

Have the class form three or four circles in the room. One student should stand in the middle of each circle. Give each group a ball. Start the music and have the groups pass the ball around the circle. When the music stops, the student in the middle gives a spelling word or curriculum question (from the list) to the student holding the ball.

If the question is answered correctly, that student goes to the middle, and the original student joins the circle. If the question is incorrect, the student is out of the game and takes a seat. The game is repeated until there is one winner in each group.

You can have one winner in each group, or when the groups get smaller, students can form one circle so there is one winner.

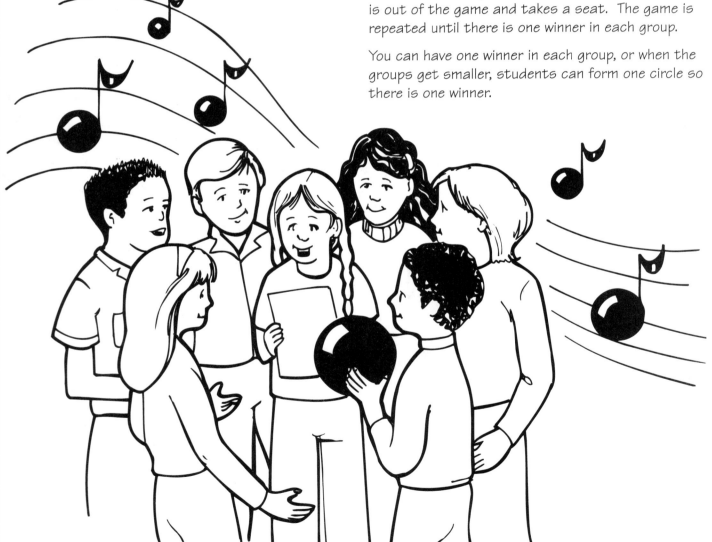

TLC10560 Copyright © Teaching & Learning Company, Carthage, IL 62321-0010

Bell Ringer

Object of the Game

Help students connect two curricular topics.

Preparation

List of words or questions

Materials

supplies for an obstacle course, a bell or buzzer

Directions

Have students build an obstacle course in the classroom. An example of the obstacle course is: a path through desks and around chairs, jump over a Hula-Hoop™, bounce a ball three times, do five jumping jacks and ring a bell (or buzzer).

Divide the class into two teams and have them line up at the chalkboard. Have one student from each team ready to write on the board. Read a question. The students race to write the correct answer on the board and travel through the obstacle course to be first to ring the bell. The winning team gets one point.

If the answer is incorrect, the student does not get to run the obstacle course. Repeat until all students have had a chance to answer.

Give an incentive to the winning team.

Game Variations

This game may be played outside. The students write their answers on a piece of paper before they run through the obstacle course.

The opposing teams must run through the obstacle course in opposite directions. Be sure to place a bell at both ends.

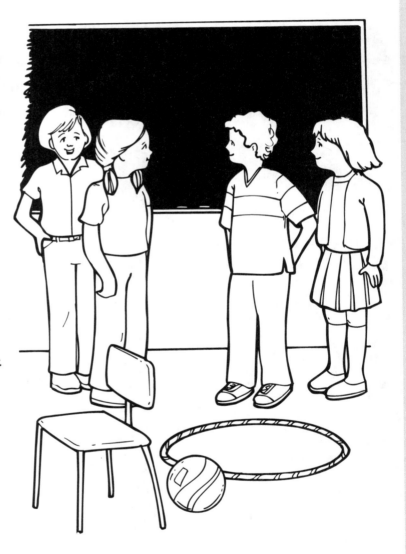

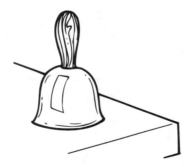

TLC10560 Copyright © Teaching & Learning Company, Carthage, IL 62321-0010

Pick and Pass

Object of the Game

Review current curriculum topics.

Preparation

List of questions

Materials

two plastic bowls, paper cut in smaller pieces

Directions

Write each student's name on a piece of paper and place them in the first plastic bowl.

Write curriculum questions on pieces of paper and place them in the second plastic bowl.

Pass both bowls to a student. The student picks a name from the first bowl and a question from the second bowl. The student whose name is drawn must answer the questions. If the student draws his or her own name, that student must answer the question.

If the student answers correctly, he or she gets the two bowls and asks a question. Play until all the students have had a turn. If the answer is incorrect, the student loses the turn and another name is picked. The new student is given the same question. Repeat the question until a correct answer is given.

Do not replace students' names in the bowl. The questions can be replaced in the bowl if necessary.

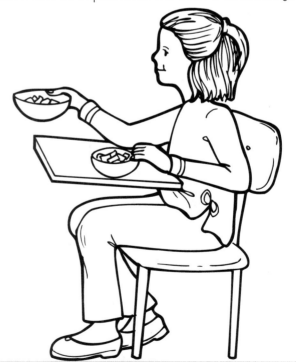

TLC10560 Copyright © Teaching & Learning Company, Carthage, IL 62321-0010

Circling the Universe

Object of the Game

Review curriculum topics.

Preparation

None

Materials

flash cards or question cards

Directions

Start with all the students sitting at their desks. The first student stands next to the desk of the student behind him or her. Flash a card. The first student who answers the question correctly moves on.

If the student standing correctly answers first, he or she moves to the desk of the next student in the row. If the student sitting answers correctly first, he or she moves on to the desk of the next student while the other student sits in that desk. The play continues until a student reaches his or her original chair, having made it all around the classroom.

Game Variations

a. The students may sit in a circle and move one person to the right.

b. A student holds the flash card or asks the question.

c. To save time, divide the class in half and have two games going at the same time.

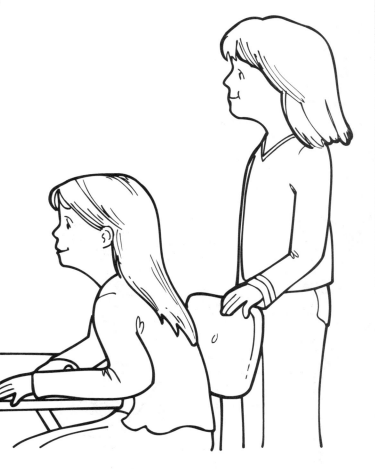

TLC10560 Copyright © Teaching & Learning Company, Carthage, IL 62321-0010

Stamp and Drum

Object of the Game

Review curriculum as a whole class.

Preparation

List of curriculum statements that can be answered "true" or "false"

Materials

None

Directions

Ask a "yes" (true) or "no" (false) question. For example, "The capital of California is Sacramento."

If the answer is "yes" (true), the students drum their desk with their fingers.

If the answer is "no" (false), the students stamp their feet on the floor.

If a student answers incorrectly and is caught, he or she is out of the game and must sit on the floor next to a desk. That student is no longer allowed to drum or stamp, but should continue to pay attention.

Game Variations

Play the game on an honor system. Students must drop out of the game and sit on the floor if they answer incorrectly. They should then write their answers instead of drumming and stamping.

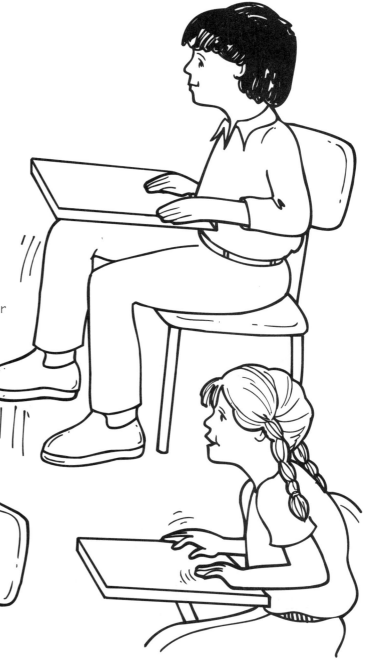

TLC10560 Copyright © Teaching & Learning Company, Carthage, IL 62321-0010

Sparkle

Object of the Game
Review spelling words or vocabulary words.

Preparation
List of words

Materials
None

Directions
Have students stand in a circle. Give a spelling word. The first student in the circle says the first letter of the word, the second student says the second letter. Continue in this manner until the word is spelled. The student in line after the word is spelled says "Sparkle," putting the next student in line out of the game.

If a student cannot give a correct letter, then he or she is out of the game. The next student in the circle must give the correct letter.

Game Variations
a. After the last letter of the word is said, the next two students race to say "Sparkle." The winner remains in the circle and the other student is out. If they say it at the same time, it is a tie and both stay in the game.

b. After the word is spelled:
- The next student in line gives an antonym or synonym for the spelling word. Then the next student in line says, "Sparkle."
- The next student in line gives the word's definition.
- The next student in line uses the word in a sentence.

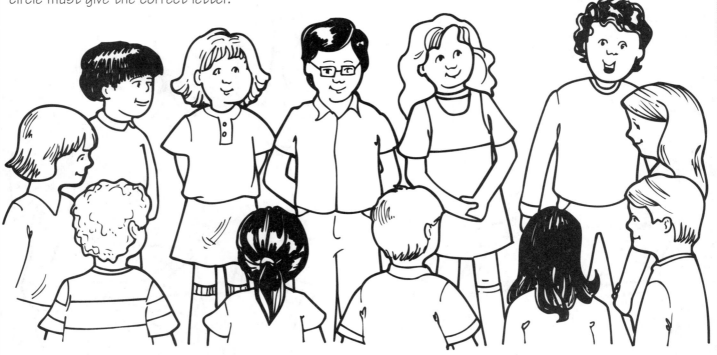

TLC10560 Copyright © Teaching & Learning Company, Carthage, IL 62321-0010

Stand Up!

Object of the Game

Review curriculum like spelling or vocabulary words.

Preparation

List of words

Materials

None

Directions

Have students stand by their seats. Give a word and point to a student who says the first letter of the word. Point to another student who gives the next letter. Repeat until the word is spelled. Continue to follow the same pattern of students. When one word is finished, give another word and continue the game. If a student gives the wrong letter, he or she sits down and is out of the game.

Rules

Do not repeat the word or last letter. Encourage students to listen.

Game Variations

After the word is spelled:

- The next student may give an antonym or synonym for the word.
- The next student gives the definition of the word.
- The next student uses the word in a sentence.

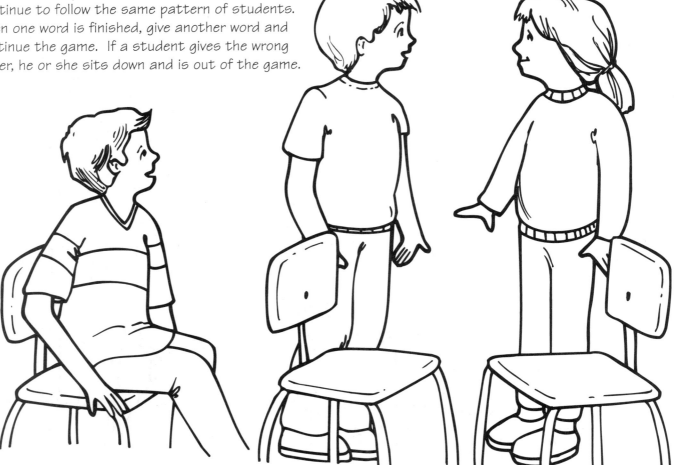

TLC10560 Copyright © Teaching & Learning Company, Carthage, IL 62321-0010

Prove You're Right

Object of the Game

Review current curriculum.

Preparation

List of curriculum questions

Materials

overhead projector, pen for overhead, paper, pencils

Directions

Separate the students into four-person teams. Make sure each team has paper and a pencil.

Have the teams take turns sending a student to the overhead. Each student must take a turn.

Give a question and have teams race to write the answer. The student at the overhead must try to beat the rest of the teams. When one of the teams is finished writing, they yell "Done!"

• If the team member at the overhead wins, that team receives two points.

• If a team wins that is not at the overhead, they receive one point.

Continue playing until every student has a turn at the overhead.

Give an incentive to the winning team.

Game Variations

a. Give a time limit to the game to encourage fast answers.

b. The first team to reach 10 points wins the game.

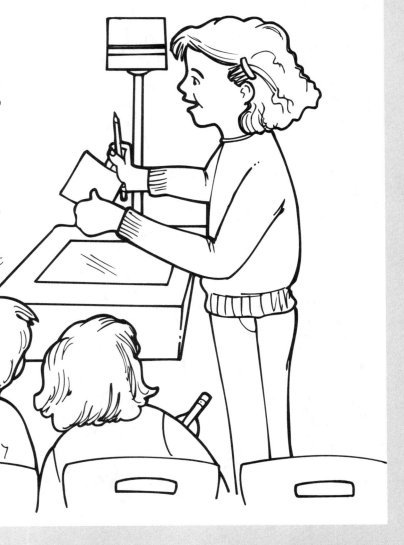

TLC10560 Copyright © Teaching & Learning Company, Carthage, IL 62321-0010

Second Chance

Object of the Game

Review current curriculum. Note: This is a good game to play outside, where there is plenty of room.

Preparation

List of curriculum questions

Materials

None

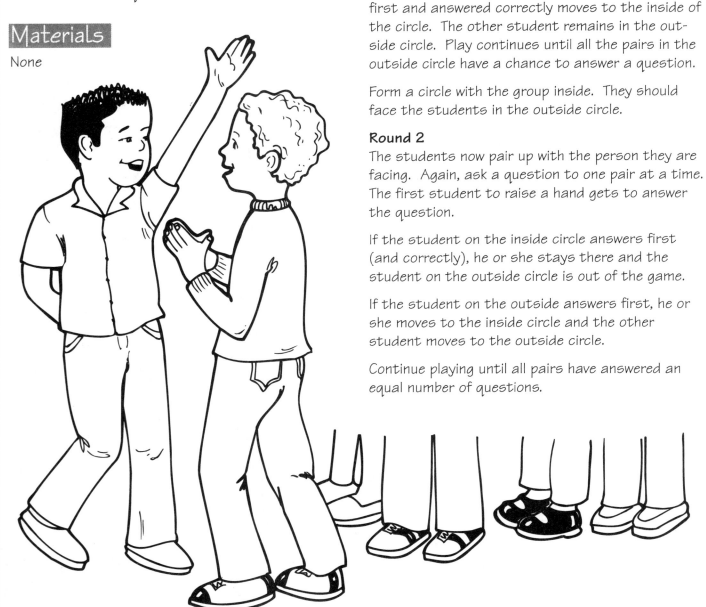

Directions

Have the class make a circle. Students should then pair up with someone next to them.

Round 1

Give a question to one pair at a time. As soon as you read the question, the two students race to raise their hand to answer. The student who was first and answered correctly moves to the inside of the circle. The other student remains in the outside circle. Play continues until all the pairs in the outside circle have a chance to answer a question.

Form a circle with the group inside. They should face the students in the outside circle.

Round 2

The students now pair up with the person they are facing. Again, ask a question to one pair at a time. The first student to raise a hand gets to answer the question.

If the student on the inside circle answers first (and correctly), he or she stays there and the student on the outside circle is out of the game.

If the student on the outside answers first, he or she moves to the inside circle and the other student moves to the outside circle.

Continue playing until all pairs have answered an equal number of questions.

TLC10560 Copyright © Teaching & Learning Company, Carthage, IL 62321-0010

Snake

Object of the Game

Review the eight parts of speech (noun, verb, adverb, adjective, pronoun, preposition, conjunction, interjection).

Preparation

None

Materials

None

Directions

The students stand by their desks. When you say "Begin," the students begin walking, following each other to form a snake that circles around the desks. Call out "Nouns!" and name a student to start.

Each student must call out a noun until five students are eliminated. A student is eliminated if he or she cannot think of a new noun or repeats one already said. Eliminated students must sit down.

Then call out "Verbs!" All students can play again. Continue through the entire list of parts of speech.

Curriculum Variations

Have students list:

- social studies facts
- science chemical terms
- states of the United States
- Presidents
- continents
- countries of the world

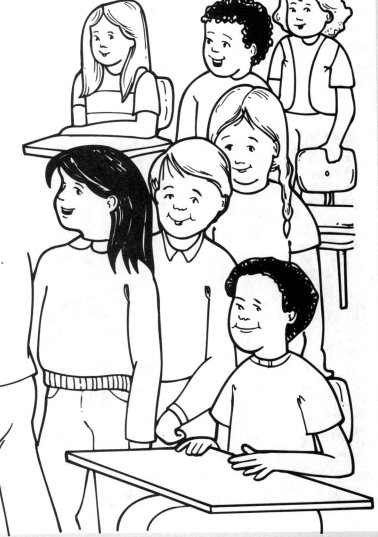

TLC10560 Copyright © Teaching & Learning Company, Carthage, IL 62321-0010

Why Use Incentives?

Learning is dependent on students being active listeners and participants in the process. It does not matter what a teacher is teaching if the students are not paying attention. Incentives can provide an environment for learning to occur. Incentives encourage students to become part of the learning process and give them a reason to remain focused.

Teaching classroom management strategy is essential for success. You must teach, discuss, model and review the strategy before beginning its use. For example, if you plan to have students earn an extra recess by writing the letters R-E-C-E-S-S on the board when students follow classroom rules and directives, you must explain what will happen, answer any questions and model how the students can earn and lose letters for a full school day.

- Model this strategy by saying things like, "Everyone got out their texts and opened to page 12 in a very short time, which earns our class the letter R." Write the letter R on the board. If the class is not working and is spending time talking, say "Our class is not working quietly on their assigned pages, therefore we lose the letter R." Then erase the letter. Make sure the students understand how to earn the letter R again, and why it was erased. When you are discussing, keep it positive and do not mention specific students' names.

- The next day, do a quick review with the students and implement the classroom management strategy by actually placing up or taking down the letters. If the students have not internalized the strategy, it will not change behaviors. The most important part of any management strategy is that all students understand how and why it works.

Although creating and preparing classroom management incentives may take some time in the beginning, the outcome will be worth it. By dedicating a small amount of time to preparing a strategy and incentive in advance, you can increase learning, raise morale and ensure a positive classroom atmosphere.

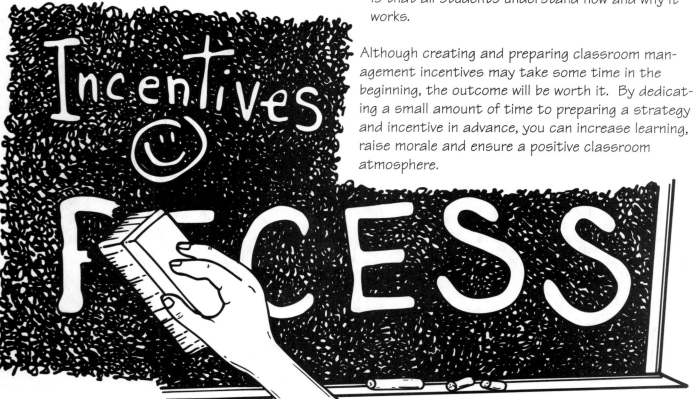

TLC10560 Copyright © Teaching & Learning Company, Carthage, IL 62321-0010

Suggestions for Incentives

No-Cost Incentives

Note: There is a generic coupon on page 55.
- Extra recess with a friend coupon
- Extra computer time coupon
- Extra time in the reading center coupon
- Extra days to complete an assignment coupon
- Extra Physical Education for the group
- No homework coupon
- Lunch inside classroom with a friend
- Lunch inside with a teacher
- Lunch with the principal
- Sit at teacher's desk for a day
- Sit in special chair for a lesson
- Free time in classroom
- Ten points added to one grade
- Chew gum in class for a day
- Opportunity to make up an assignment
- Drop lowest assignment grade
- Bring a game from home to play with a friend
- Wear pajamas to school for a day
- Bring a snack and eat it during class
- Be the teacher for a subject
- Visit the art center for an hour
- Visit the media center for an hour
- Line leader for a day
- Work with a friend for a day
- Choose the next game
- Listen to music during free time
- Read a story to the class
- Wear a hat for a day
- Be leader for a day
- Watch a movie
- Take home an award certificate

Other Incentives

- pencils
- erasers
- notebooks
- books
- bags of chips
- ribbons
- candy

Other Options

- Hold a weekly auction where students can use their incentive tokens/tickets to bid on items.
- Weekly have a store where students can purchase items with their incentive tokens/tickets.
- Offer students a bank. They can deposit tokens/tickets and earn interest by leaving them in the bank. By leaving one token in for one week, the student will get two. (To help facilitate this, see the Bank Tracking Sheet on page 56.)

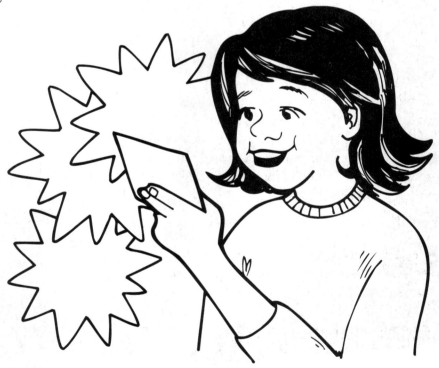

Classroom Management Strategies

Incentives Linked to Curriculum

Any form of classroom incentive should be associated with the curriculum in the classroom. There are several examples. It is easiest to link incentive programs to social studies and science topics; however, any subject can be used. Just link any key phrase or idea to the incentive program. You can type it in a special font or print it on a unique color of paper. Students work to earn these tickets, tokens, coupons.

Cut out the phrases and keep them handy. If you plan to reuse the incentives, they should be laminated. If the incentives will only be used once, have students put their names on them when they have earned them.

Use these incentives to increase desired behaviors and reward students. If students are not participating, hold the container, take out a token and ask for a desired response. If a student participates, continue teaching while walking to the student's desk and dropping an incentive on the desk. Do not take away from the momentum of the lesson, but reinforce positive behavior in the classroom.

If a student is demonstrating undesirable behaviors such as talking during a lesson, you can also use an incentive to thank a student in the same area. Be sure to thank the rewarded student for working quietly. This can be done quickly without interrupting the lesson.

Here are some suggestions for incentive programs.

Communities

Students can earn tickets for positive community behavior. Tickets can list common community helpers, like police officers, fire fighters, nurses, teachers, etc.

Revolutionary War

Students earn tax tokens related to King George III taxing the colonists. Students with desired behaviors are rewarded like Loyalists, and students pay taxes for things that they need to do such as a Navigation Tax to move around the room and sharpen pencil or use the restroom, a Stamp Tax to turn in a paper where students use a rubber stamp to put on a paper and pay to turn it in, etc. Students also pay tax when exhibiting an undesirable behavior. (See sample tax tokens on page 57.)

Westward Movement in the United States

Students can earn Manifest Destiny tickets for positive behavior. See page 58.

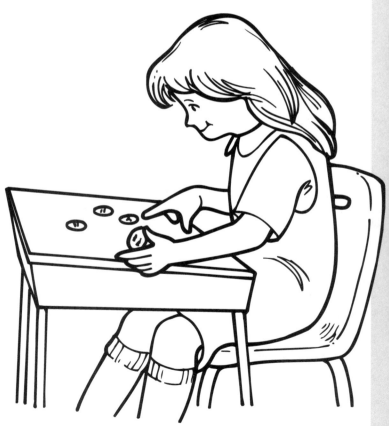

TLC10560 Copyright © Teaching & Learning Company, Carthage, IL 62321-0010

Classroom Management Strategies

Gold Rush

Hide gold rocks or tokens around the room. Students can find and collect them. Students may look for gold at only specified times. Time is earned through good behavior. You can also allow students to spend their other incentives to buy time to hunt for gold. Students lose incentives if they look for gold outside of the designated time.

World Countries

Students can earn tickets based on the wealth of countries of the world. The goal is for a student to earn a certain number of the poorer country tickets to trade for a wealthier country ticket. Once a number of wealthier country tickets are earned, the student can purchase something on the incentive list.

Solar System

Students can earn stars for good behavior. They can work to collect enough to complete a constellation that they can trade for an incentive. See page 59.

Math Is Power

Students earn tickets to trade for bigger incentives. You could also hold a daily drawing for students who do not want to save their tickets. See page 60.

Drawings

Daily, weekly and monthly drawings will get students excited about earning the classroom incentive. Have a collection container for the incentives. Be sure students include their names when they enter the drawing.

You can empty daily drawing slips each day into a weekly drawing container. Weekly drawing slips can also be kept for a monthly drawing. Daily prizes are small, weekly prizes are a bit bigger, and monthly prizes are big. Daily drawing prizes can be a small eraser, a small lollipop or being the first person to line up that day. Weekly drawings can include a 15-minute computer time coupon, a candy bar or a free time coupon. Monthly drawings can include a homework coupon, lunch inside with friends coupon or an extra credit points coupon.

Always tell students in advance when the drawings will be conducted and what the prizes are. It is best to switch up the prizes to keep students interested.

Spinner

Students can save their incentives for a chance to use the spinner. Students trade in the incentives for two spins, either twice on one side or once on each side. See pages 61-62.

Group Competitions

You can motivate students and build class unity with competitive incentives. Linking group competitions to curriculum is an excellent way for students to review and focus on specific subjects. On the following page are examples of some group competitions.

TLC10560 Copyright © Teaching & Learning Company, Carthage, IL 62321-0010

Classroom Management Strategies

Civil War

Place students in two teams, the North and the South. Place a poster board at the front of the room with a T-chart on it. Points are awarded when students on either side exhibit desired behaviors. Use this for a week or more and see which side wins.

Clowning Around

Create groups with four, five or six students. Color-code the groups. Make a chart, like the one on page 63, on poster board and place it at the front of the room. Number each group and write the numbers in the center of the poster board. Add plus signs to one side of each number and negative signs to the other side. Place a clown from page 64 over the number for each group. Move each group's clown according to desired or undesired behaviors.

If a group gets to the end of the negative side, they must spend recess inside. At the end of the week, the group whose clown is closest to the end of the positive side receives an incentive. Then form students in new groups for the next week.

Table Points

Group students in fours, fives or sixes. Allow 10 minutes for each to make a sign with their group name. Place it in the center of their desks. Write the group names on poster board. Give points to teams that are exhibiting desired behaviors. Don't take away points, instead give points to all other tables when one table is exhibiting undesirable behaviors. At the end of the week, the team with the most points receives an incentive. Then form new groups.

R-E-C-E-S-S

Students earn the letters by exhibiting desired behaviors. The incentive is only earned if the class works together. When the students earn a letter, write it on the board. Letters can be erased when the class is not exhibiting desired behaviors. When the class spells the whole word, they get an extra recess. The class can spell other words like *ice cream party, extra P.E.* or *special walk*.

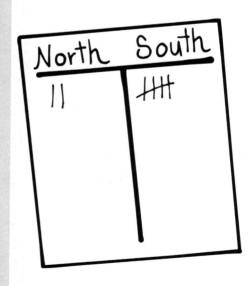

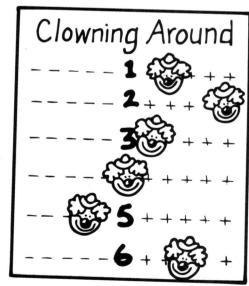

TLC10560 Copyright © Teaching & Learning Company, Carthage, IL 62321-0010

Incentive Coupons

_____
(Type of Coupon)

_____
(Student's Signature)

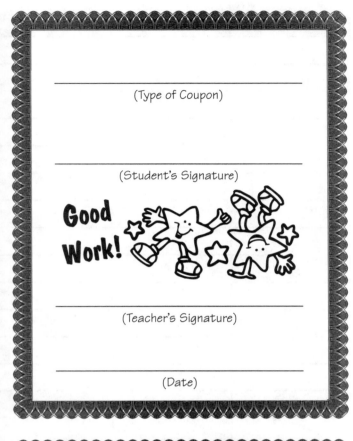

_____
(Teacher's Signature)

_____
(Date)

_____
(Type of Coupon)

_____
(Student's Signature)

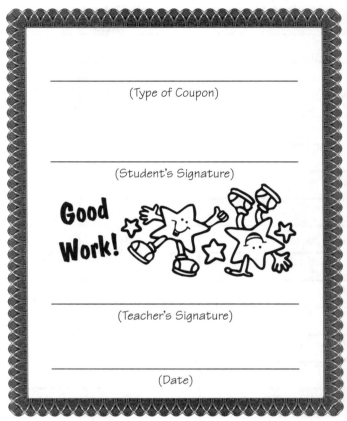

_____
(Teacher's Signature)

_____
(Date)

_____
(Type of Coupon)

_____
(Student's Signature)

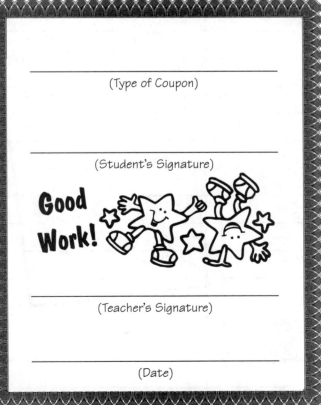

_____
(Teacher's Signature)

_____
(Date)

_____
(Type of Coupon)

_____
(Student's Signature)

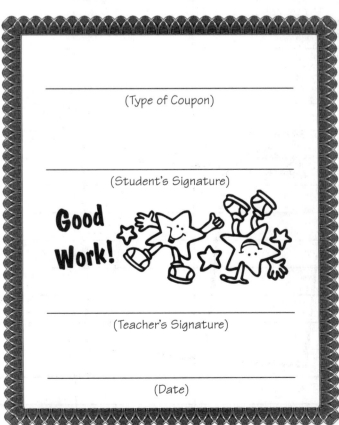

_____
(Teacher's Signature)

_____
(Date)

TLC10560 Copyright © Teaching & Learning Company, Carthage, IL 62321-0010

Bank Tracking Sheet

Student Name	Deposit Date	Deposit Date	Deposit Date	Deposit Date	Total
1.					
2.					
3.					
4.					
5.					
6.					
7.					
8.					
9.					
10.					
11.					
12.					
13.					
14.					
15.					
16.					
17.					
18.					
19.					
20.					
21.					
22.					
23.					
24.					
25.					
26.					
27.					
28.					
29.					
30.					

TLC10560 Copyright © Teaching & Learning Company, Carthage, IL 62321-0010

Tax Tokens

 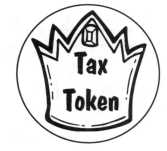  

  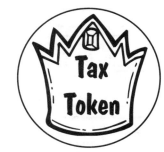 

TLC10560 Copyright © Teaching & Learning Company, Carthage, IL 62321-0010

Manifest Destiny Tickets

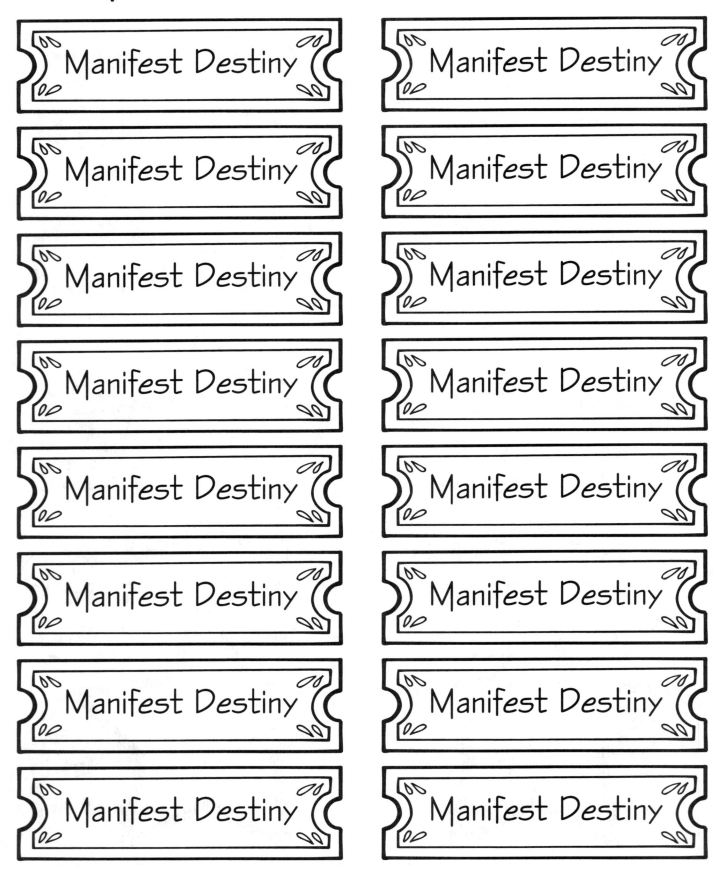

TLC10560 Copyright © Teaching & Learning Company, Carthage, IL 62321-0010

Solar System Stars

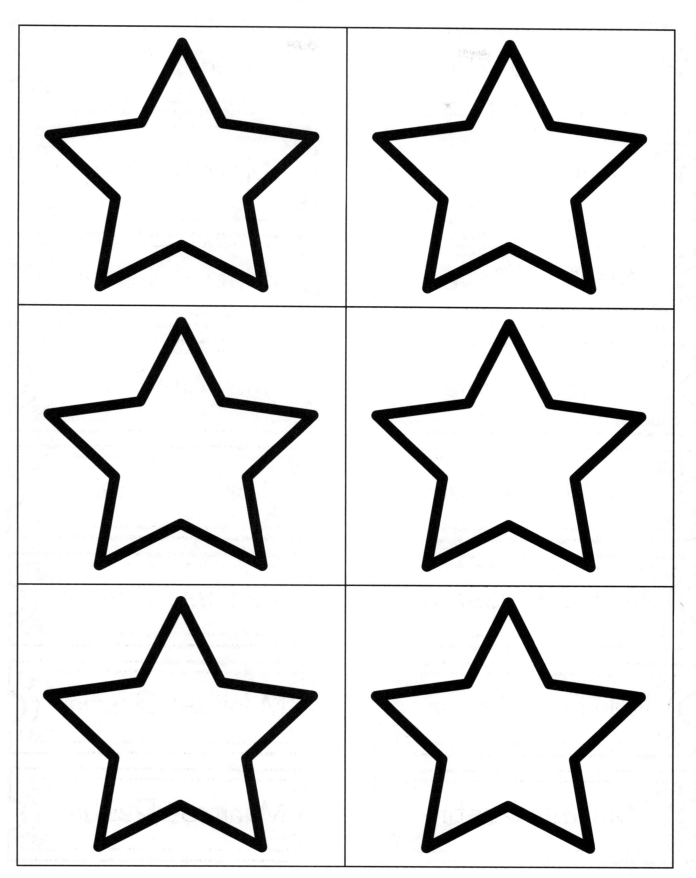

Math Is Power Tickets

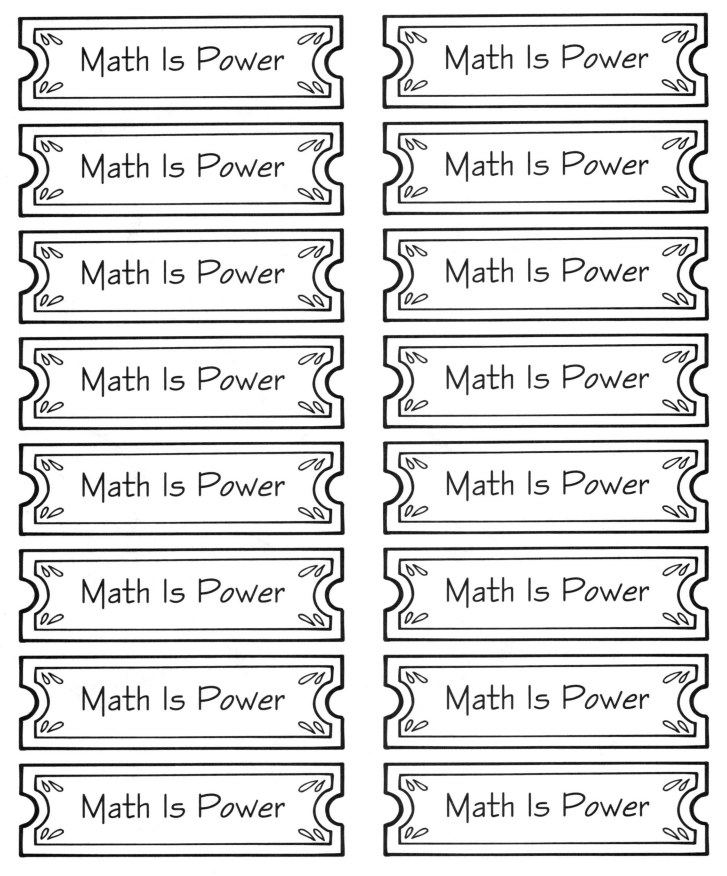

TLC10560 Copyright © Teaching & Learning Company, Carthage, IL 62321-0010

Spinner Incentive

(Can be copied back to back with page 62.)

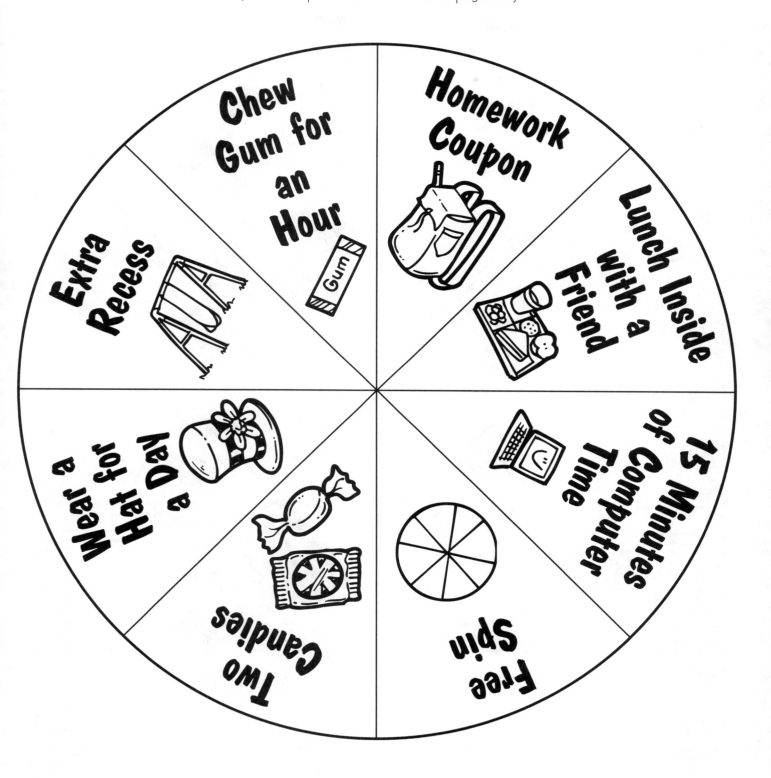

Spinner Incentive

(Can be copied back to back with page 61.)

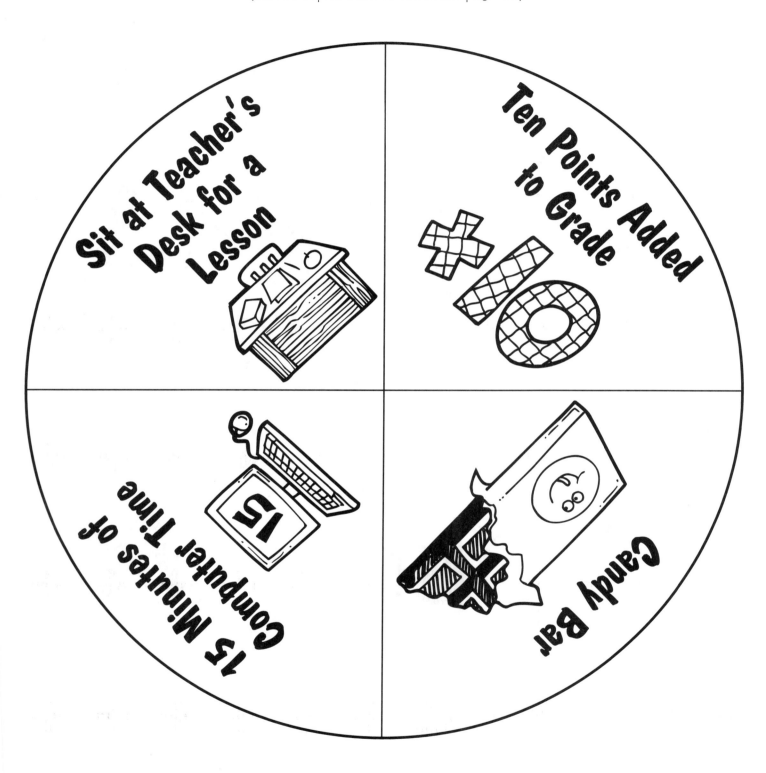

TLC10560 Copyright © Teaching & Learning Company, Carthage, IL 62321-0010

Clowning Around Chart

- - - - - - - 1 + + + + + +

- - - - - - - 2 + + + + + +

- - - - - - - 3 + + + + + +

- - - - - - - 4 + + + + + +

- - - - - - - 5 + + + + + +

- - - - - - - 6 + + + + + +

TLC10560 Copyright © Teaching & Learning Company, Carthage, IL 62321-0010

Clowning Around

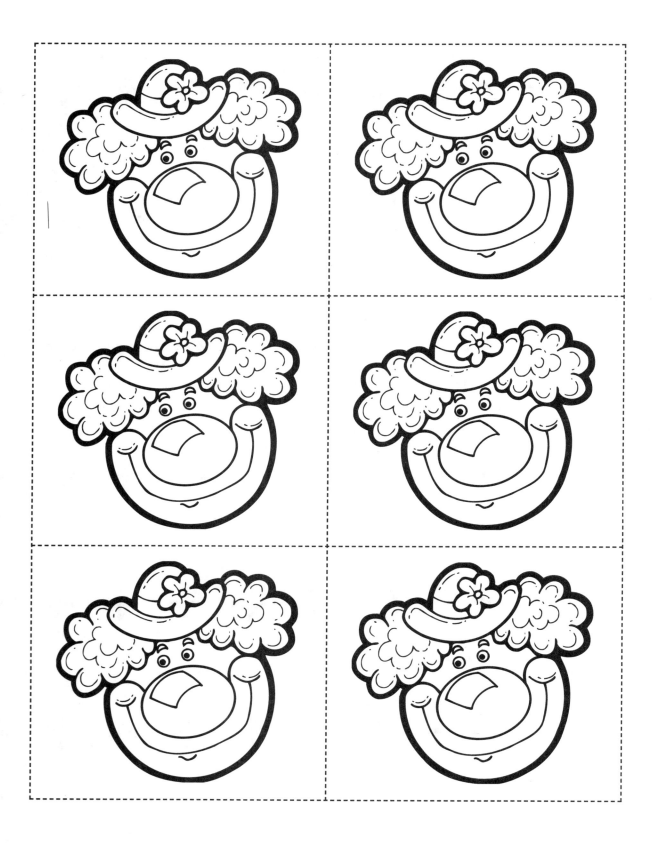

TLC10560 Copyright © Teaching & Learning Company, Carthage, IL 62321-0010